Beginner's Guide To Calisthenics

An Ultimate Workouts Guide For Building Strength Regardless Of Your Fitness Level

Vicky Klocko

Table of Contents

CHAPTER ONE

Introduction

Calisthenics is a form of exercise that uses bodyweight movements to build strength, flexibility, and endurance. It's a versatile and accessible way to get fit without the need for equipment, although sometimes simple items like bars or rings might be used.

Core Principles

Bodyweight Exercises: The core of calisthenics involves exercises like push-ups, pull-ups, dips, squats, lunges, and planks.

Progressive Overload: Increasing the challenge gradually by modifying exercises or increasing repetitions.

Full-Body Engagement: Most calisthenics exercises engage multiple muscle groups, promoting holistic fitness.

Functional Strength: Focuses on movements that mimic real-life activities, improving overall functionality.

Flexibility and Mobility: Many calisthenics exercises involve stretching and movements that improve flexibility and mobility.

Basic Exercises

Push-Ups: Strengthen chest, shoulders, and triceps.

Pull-Ups/Chin-Ups: Work the back, arms, and core.

Dips: Target the triceps, chest, and shoulders.

Squats/Lunges: Develop lower body strength.

Planks: Engage core muscles for stability.

Advanced Moves

Muscle-Ups: A combination of a pull-up and a dip, requiring explosive strength.

Handstands: Develop balance, shoulder, and core strength.

Planche: Advanced move where the body is held parallel to the ground, demanding immense upper body strength.

Human Flag: Sideways hold on a vertical pole, testing core and upper body strength.

What Makes Calisthenics Unique?

Minimal Equipment: Unlike traditional weight training, calisthenics primarily uses bodyweight, making it accessible anywhere.

Functional Strength: Emphasizes movements that mimic real-life activities, enhancing overall functionality.

Versatility: Offers a wide range of exercises, from beginner to advanced, allowing progression without the need for additional equipment.

Focus on Control and Balance: Many exercises require control of body movements, fostering better coordination and balance.

Adaptability: Suitable for all fitness levels, with exercises that can be modified to challenge both beginners and seasoned athletes.

Benefits of Bodyweight Training

Strength Development: Builds lean muscle and functional strength without the need for heavy weights.

Improved Flexibility: Many calisthenics exercises involve dynamic movements that promote flexibility.

Enhanced Body Control: Develops better coordination, balance, and proprioception.

Increased Mobility: Encourages a wider range of motion, aiding in joint health.

Accessible and Cost-Effective: Minimal equipment needed, making it accessible to most people without a significant financial investment.

Getting Started Mindset

Patience and Consistency: Progress in calisthenics takes time. Focus on consistent practice rather than immediate results.

Embrace Challenges: Understand that initial exercises might be difficult, but they provide a platform for improvement.

Listen to Your Body: Pay attention to your body's signals. Rest and recovery are crucial for progress and injury prevention.

Set Realistic Goals: Establish achievable short-term and long-term goals to track your progress and maintain motivation.

Celebrate Small Wins: Every step forward, no matter how small, is a victory. Acknowledge and celebrate your progress along the way.

Starting calisthenics requires a blend of patience, determination, and a willingness to challenge yourself. It's a journey that rewards dedication and consistency, offering numerous physical and mental benefits while allowing you to sculpt your body and abilities using

your own strength.

CHAPTER TWO

Types of Calisthenics

Calisthenics encompasses various types and methods, each focusing on different aspects of strength, flexibility, and skill development. Here are some prominent types and methods within the realm of calisthenics:

Basic Calisthenics: Involves fundamental bodyweight exercises like push-ups, pull-ups, squats, lunges, and planks. These exercises form the foundation for more advanced movements.

Street Workout/Bar Calisthenics: Often performed in outdoor spaces or with street workout equipment like pull-up bars and parallel bars. Emphasizes freestyle movements, creative combinations, and often includes impressive static and dynamic exercises.

Gymnastic Calisthenics: Influenced by gymnastics, it focuses on advanced bodyweight movements such as planches, handstands, and muscle-ups. Requires high levels of strength, balance, and body control.

Weighted Calisthenics: Integrates additional weight, such as weight vests or ankle weights, into bodyweight exercises to increase resistance and challenge.

Skill-Based Calisthenics: Concentrates on developing specific skills like hand balancing, human flags, or levers, requiring mastery of complex movements and techniques.

Methods/Styles Used in Calisthenics

Progressive Overload: Increasing the difficulty of exercises gradually to stimulate muscle growth and strength development.

Isometric Training: Involves static positions that build strength in specific muscle groups without joint movement, like holding a plank or a static handstand.

Plyometrics: Utilizes explosive movements to improve power and speed, often seen in exercises like plyometric push-ups or jump squats.

Circuit Training: Combines different calisthenics exercises into a high-intensity circuit, targeting various muscle groups while enhancing cardiovascular fitness.

High-Volume Training: Focuses on performing a high number of repetitions of a particular exercise to build muscular endurance.

Skill Progressions: Breaks down complex movements into smaller, achievable progressions, allowing individuals to gradually build up to mastering advanced skills.

Each method and style within calisthenics offers its own unique benefits, whether it's building strength, achieving new skills, or enhancing overall fitness. Choosing the right method often depends on individual goals, preferences, and current fitness levels.

Push-Ups and Variations

Basic Push-Up:

- Targets chest, shoulders, and triceps.

- Start in a plank position, lower your body by bending elbows, then push back up.

Variations:

- **Wide-Arm Push-Up:** Hands placed wider than shoulder-width apart, emphasizing chest muscles.

- **Diamond Push-Up:** Hands close together forming a diamond shape, targeting triceps.

- **Decline Push-Up:** Feet elevated, adding more resistance.

- **One-Arm Push-Up:** Advanced variation, performed with one hand behind the back.

Bodyweight Squats:

- Targets quadriceps, hamstrings, and glutes.

- Stand with feet shoulder-width apart, squat down by bending knees and hips, then return to standing.

Lunges:

- Works quadriceps, hamstrings, glutes, and calves.
- Step forward with one leg, lower your hips until both knees are bent at a 90-degree angle, then return to standing.

Variations:

- **Jump Squats:** Incorporates explosiveness into squats by jumping at the top of the movement.

- **Split Squats:** Stationary lunges focusing more on one leg at a time.

Pull-Ups:

- Engages back, biceps, and shoulders.

- Hang from a bar with palms facing away, pull body up until chin clears the bar, and then lower back down.

Rows (Horizontal Pull):

- Works back muscles and biceps.

- Using a bar or rings, position yourself under it and pull your chest toward the bar, keeping your body straight.

Variations:

- **Chin-Ups:** Palms facing towards you, emphasizing biceps.

- **L-Sit Pull-Ups:** Performed with legs extended in an L-shape, targeting core and upper body.

- **Inverted Rows:** Performed on a lower bar or rings, body at an angle, pulling up similar to a rowing motion.

Core Strengthening with Planks:

Plank:

- Engages core muscles for stability.

- Hold a push-up position with elbows on the ground, body straight from head to heels.

Variations:

- **Side Plank:** Support body on one forearm, body in a straight line, engaging obliques.

- **Plank with Leg Lifts:** From a plank position, lift one leg off the ground while maintaining core stability.

- **Plank Rotations:** Transition from a regular plank to side planks, alternating sides.

Mastering these fundamental exercises and their variations lays a solid foundation for a comprehensive calisthenics routine. They target multiple muscle groups, providing a balanced approach to strength and conditioning. As you progress, you can gradually increase difficulty or try more advanced variations to keep challenging your body.

CHAPTER THREE
Progressions and Technique Refinement

Advancing Push-Up Variations:

- Focus on mastering the basic push-up with proper form before progressing to variations.

- Gradually increase repetitions and ensure a full range of motion.

Progressive Variations:

- Once basic push-ups are mastered, advance to wide-arm push-ups, then diamond push-ups, gradually challenging different muscle groups.

- Try decline push-ups by elevating feet on a stable surface for increased difficulty.

Strength Building Techniques:

- Slow down the tempo to increase time under tension, emphasizing muscle engagement.

- Add explosive power with plyometric push-ups by pushing off the ground forcefully.

Perfecting Pull-Up Form:

- Ensure a firm grip on the bar with hands slightly wider than shoulder-width apart.

- Maintain a straight body from head to heels without swinging or arching the back excessively.

Full Range of Motion:

- Start from a dead hang, fully extend arms at the bottom, then pull yourself up until your chin clears the bar.

- Lower yourself in a controlled manner to the dead hang position without dropping suddenly.

Assisted Pull-Ups and Negatives:

- Use resistance bands or an assisted pull-up machine to reduce bodyweight and work on proper form.

- Focus on eccentric (negative) pull-ups by slowing down the lowering phase to build strength.

Increasing Lower Body Strength:

- Once bodyweight squats are comfortable, progress to jump squats for explosive power.

- Add weight with a backpack, holding a weight plate, or using a barbell for added resistance.

Lunges and Their Progressions:

- Incorporate walking lunges, reverse lunges, or jumping lunges for variety and challenge.

- Utilize split squats or Bulgarian split squats to isolate each leg and increase difficulty.

Core Exercise Progressions:

- Gradually increase plank duration and focus on maintaining proper form throughout.

- Move to more challenging variations like side planks, plank with leg lifts, or plank rotations.

Dynamic Core Exercises:

- Introduce dynamic movements like mountain climbers, bicycle crunches, or Russian twists to engage the core dynamically.

Advanced Core Movements:

- Progress to exercises like hanging leg raises, dragon flags, or hollow body holds for increased core strength.

Remember, progression in calisthenics is about gradual and controlled advancement. Focus on proper form, gradually increase difficulty, and listen to your body to prevent injury. Consistency and patience are key to mastering these progressions and refining technique in calisthenics exercises.

Importance of Consistency

Progress Requires Regularity: Consistent practice allows your body to adapt and improve gradually.

Skill Refinement: Regular repetition of exercises hones technique and form, essential for progression.

Muscle Memory: Consistency builds muscle memory, enhancing performance and reducing the risk of injury.

Mental Adaptation: Consistent workouts establish a routine and develop discipline, fostering a strong mental attitude.

Establishing A Solid Routine

Balanced Approach: Include exercises targeting all major muscle groups for a comprehensive workout.

Progressive Overload: Gradually increase intensity, repetitions, or difficulty to challenge your muscles and promote growth.

Rest and Recovery: Incorporate rest days to allow muscles to repair and grow stronger. Overtraining can hinder progress.

Adaptability: Modify your routine as needed, considering factors like fitness goals, available time, and personal preferences.

CHAPTER FOUR
Understanding Muscle Engagement

Mind-Muscle Connection: Focus on engaging the specific muscles targeted by each exercise.

Form and Technique: Proper form ensures effective muscle engagement and reduces the risk of injury.

Concentric and Eccentric Phases: Understand and control both phases of muscle contraction—shortening (concentric) and lengthening (eccentric)—for optimal development.

Isolation vs. Compound Movements:
Know when to incorporate isolated exercises for specific muscles and compound movements for overall strength.

Nutrition and Recovery in Calisthenics

Nutrition and recovery play crucial roles in maximizing performance and progress in calisthenics.

Role of Nutrition in Bodyweight Training:

Fueling Workouts: Adequate nutrition provides the energy needed for training sessions.

Muscle Repair and Growth: Protein intake supports muscle recovery and growth after workouts.

Macro and Micro Nutrients: Balancing carbohydrates, proteins, fats, vitamins, and minerals aids overall health and performance.

Hydration: Proper hydration is essential for optimal muscle function and overall performance during workouts.

Recovery Strategies for Optimal Performance

Rest and Sleep: Allow for sufficient rest between workouts and aim for quality sleep to facilitate recovery.

Active Recovery: Light exercises, yoga, or stretching sessions on rest days promote blood flow and aid recovery without excessive strain.

Nutrient Timing: Consume protein and carbohydrates after workouts to support muscle repair and replenish glycogen stores.

Foam Rolling and Stretching: Aid in muscle recovery and flexibility, reducing soreness and improving range of motion.

Balancing Diet and Exercise

Caloric Intake: Ensure a balance between energy expended during workouts and calories consumed for muscle repair and growth.

Protein Intake: Consume adequate protein to support muscle repair and growth. Aim for a balanced intake throughout the day.

Healthy Fats and Carbs: Include sources of healthy fats and complex carbohydrates for sustained energy and overall health.

Timing Meals: Consider pre-workout and post-workout meals to optimize energy levels and recovery.

Practical Tips

Meal Planning: Plan balanced meals that include a variety of nutrients to support your training regimen.

Hydration: Stay adequately hydrated throughout the day, not just during workouts.

Listen to Your Body: Pay attention to hunger cues, energy levels, and how your body responds to different foods and timing.

Injury Prevention and Safety

Absolutely, injury prevention and safety are crucial aspects of any fitness regimen, including calisthenics. Here's how you can reduce the risk of common injuries and prioritize safety:

Common Injuries and Prevention Tips:

Muscle Strains and Sprains:

Prevention: Warm up before workouts, gradually increase intensity, and incorporate dynamic stretches.

Shoulder Injuries (Rotator Cuff Strains):

Prevention: Focus on proper shoulder positioning during exercises, avoid excessive swinging or jerking motions.

Wrist and Elbow Strains:

Prevention: Ensure proper wrist alignment during exercises, avoid excessive stress on wrists, and gradually progress in advanced movements.

Lower Back Strains:

Prevention: Maintain good posture, engage core muscles properly during exercises, and avoid overextending the back.

Overuse Injuries:

Prevention: Allow for adequate rest between workouts, vary exercises to prevent repetitive stress on specific muscles or joints.

Proper Form and Technique:

Focus on Form: Prioritize proper form over the number of repetitions. Incorrect form can lead to injuries.

Gradual Progression: Start with basic exercises, master proper form, and gradually advance to more challenging movements.

Educate Yourself: Seek guidance from trainers, online resources, or instructional videos to understand correct techniques.

Listening to Your Body:

Recognize Pain vs. Discomfort: Sharp, persistent pain during or after an exercise might indicate an issue. Discomfort or muscle soreness is normal but should not be excessive or sharp.

Rest and Recovery: Allow your body time to recover between workouts. Don't push through significant pain; it might worsen an injury.

Modify as Needed: If an exercise causes discomfort or pain, modify it or seek alternatives instead of pushing through.

Practical Tips:

Warm-Up and Cool Down: Begin workouts with a dynamic warm-up and end with static stretching to improve flexibility and reduce injury risk.

Cross-Training: Incorporate different types of exercises to avoid overuse of specific muscles or joints.

Use Proper Equipment: Ensure equipment, such as bars or mats, is in good condition and suitable for your workouts.

Prioritizing safety in calisthenics involves understanding potential injury risks, focusing on proper technique, and listening to your body's signals. By gradually progressing, prioritizing form, and taking care to prevent overuse or strain, you can significantly reduce the risk of injuries during your calisthenics practice.

CHAPTER FIVE

Full Body Beginner Workout Routine

Warm-Up:

- Jumping Jacks: 2 sets of 20 reps
- Arm Circles: 2 sets of 15 reps (forward and backward)
- Bodyweight Squats: 2 sets of 15 reps

Main Workout:

- Push-Ups: 3 sets of 8-10 reps
- Bodyweight Squats: 3 sets of 10-12 reps

- Bent Knee Leg Raises (for core): 3 sets of 10-12 reps

- Assisted Pull-Ups or Inverted Rows: 3 sets of 6-8 reps

Cooldown:

- Standing Forward Fold: Hold for 30 seconds

- Cobra Stretch: Hold for 30 seconds

- Seated Forward Fold: Hold for 30 seconds

Upper Body Focus Routine:

Warm-Up:

- Arm Circles: 2 sets of 15 reps (forward and backward)

- Wrist Circles: 2 sets of 10 reps (clockwise and counterclockwise)

- Jumping Jacks: 2 sets of 20 reps

Main Workout:

- Push-Ups: 4 sets of 8-12 reps

- Assisted Pull-Ups: 4 sets of 6-8 reps

- Diamond Push-Ups: 3 sets of 6-8 reps

- Plank: 3 sets of 30-45 seconds

Cooldown:

- Shoulder Stretch: Hold for 30 seconds each arm

- Triceps Stretch: Hold for 30 seconds each arm

- Neck Stretch: Hold for 30 seconds each side

Lower Body and Core Emphasis Routine:

Warm-Up:

- Leg Swings: 2 sets of 10 reps each leg

- Hip Circles: 2 sets of 10 reps (clockwise and counterclockwise)

- Jumping Jacks: 2 sets of 20 reps

Main Workout:

- Bodyweight Squats: 4 sets of 10-15 reps

- Lunges (Forward or Reverse): 3 sets of 8-10 reps each leg

- Russian Twists: 3 sets of 12-15 reps (with or without weight)

- Plank with Leg Lifts: 3 sets of 10-12 reps (each leg)

Cooldown:

- Hamstring Stretch: Hold for 30 seconds each leg

- Quadriceps Stretch: Hold for 30 seconds each leg

- Cat-Cow Stretch: Perform for 1 minute

These sample workouts provide a foundation for beginners to start their calisthenics journey. Remember to maintain proper form, gradually increase intensity, and listen to your body. Adjust repetitions and sets based on your fitness level, and always warm up before and cool down after each session to prevent injury.

Embracing the Calisthenics Lifestyle

Embracing the calisthenics lifestyle opens doors to holistic fitness, strength, and a sense of accomplishment. Here's how to continue this journey:

Consistency and Persistence: Understand that progress takes time and consistent effort. Embrace the process and enjoy the journey.

Mind-Body Connection: Calisthenics isn't just about physical strength but also mental discipline and body awareness. Embrace the mind-body connection in your workouts.

Healthy Lifestyle: Complement your calisthenics training with a balanced diet, sufficient sleep, and stress management. These factors contribute to overall well-being and performance.

Versatility and Adaptability: Embrace the versatility of calisthenics - it can be practiced anywhere, anytime. Use this flexibility to integrate it seamlessly into your lifestyle.

THE END